Cookie, Cupcakes & Desserts

The Keto Baking Cookbook for Every Occasion

RoyalKeto

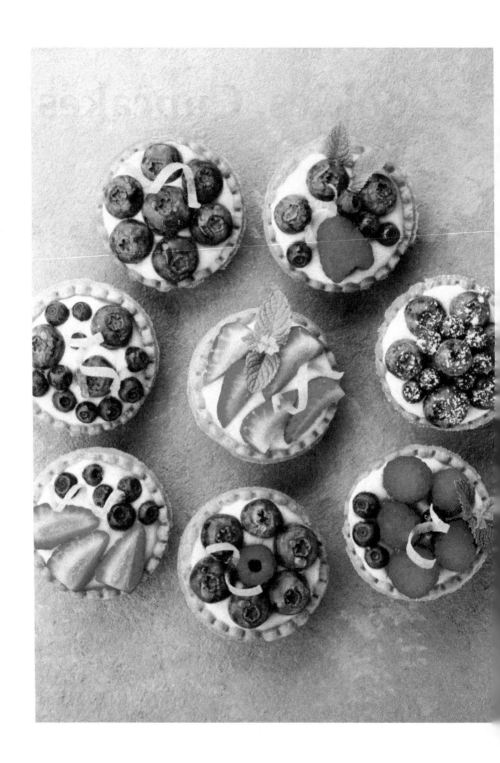

way be considered an endorsement from the trademark
holder.

Almond Butter Cup Cookies

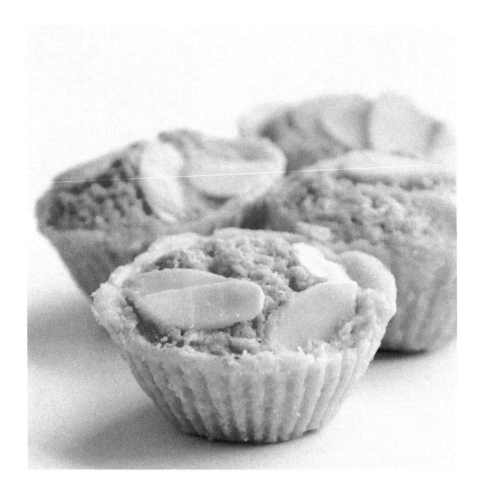

Serving: 4

Prep Time: 10 minutes

Cook Time: 90 minutes

Ingredients

- 1 teaspoon vanilla bean extract
- ¼ teaspoon almond extract

- 2 whole eggs
- ½ cup almond flour, blanched
- 2 tablespoons coconut flour
- 1 cup almond butter
- ½ cup coconut crystals
- ¼ teaspoon salt
- 1 cup dark chocolate, chopped, unsweetened

How To

1. Pre-heat your oven to 350 degree F

2. Prepare baking sheet by lightly greasing it with coconut oil

3. Add crystal, almond butter, eggs, almond extract and vanilla extract in a medium bowl

4. Mix well

5. Take another bowl and add flours, salt and mix

6. Add the flour mix to the bowl with wet ingredients and stir until combined

7. Form golf ball sized cookies and form them into peanut butter cups

8. Place cookies on baking sheet and let them bake for 12 minutes

9. Chill for 30 minutes in refrigerators

10. Melt chocolate over medium heat in double boiler and cool for 15 minutes, pour chocolate over chilled cookies

11. Serve and enjoy!

Nutrition (Per Serving)

- Calories: 163
- Fat: 10g
- Carbohydrates: 4g
- Protein: 5g

Macadamia Fat Bomb

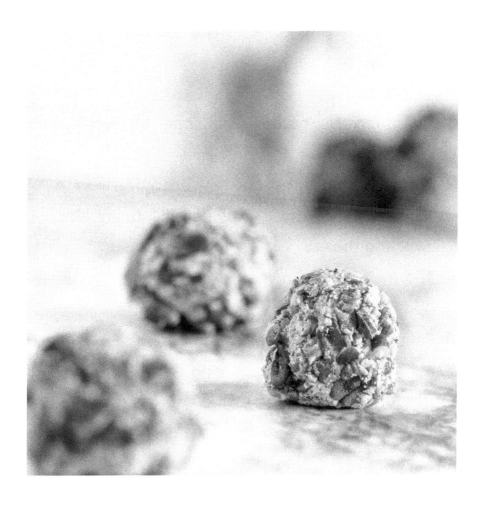

Serving: 4

Prep Time: 10 minutes + 30-60 minutes chill time

<u>**Ingredients**</u>

- 2 oz of unsweetened cocoa butter

- 4 oz of macadamia, chopped
- ¼ c of heavy cream
- 2 tbsp of unsweetened cocoa powder
- 2 tbsp of Swerve

How To

1. Melt in cocoa butter in a small saucepan over medium heat
2. Add cocoa powder to the saucepan
3. Add swerve, mix well until ingredients are blended well and melted
4. Add macadamias and stir
5. Add cream, mix and heat it up
6. Pour the mixture into Fat Bomb molds
7. Let it chill until hardened, and enjoy!

Nutrition (Per Serving)

- Calories: 247
- Fat: 23g
- Carbohydrates: 5g
- Protein: 3g

Double Berry Ice Pops

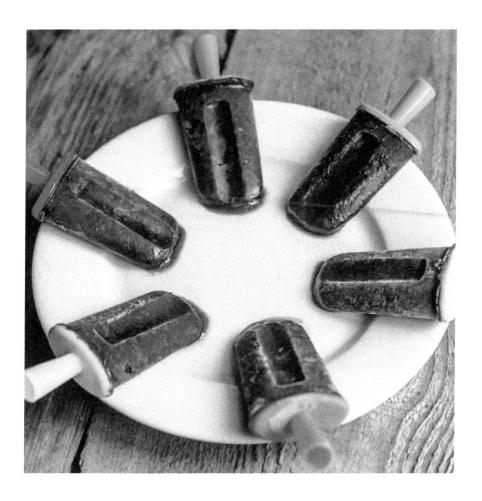

Serving: 4

Prep Time: 10 minutes + 2 hours chill time

Ingredients

- ½ tsp of vanilla extract
- ¼ c of mixed blueberries and blackberries

- ½ can use coconut cream
- ¾ c of unsweetened full-fat coconut milk
- 2 drops liquid stevia

How To

1. Take a food processor and add coconut cream, vanilla, and sweetener
2. Process well and add mixed berries, pulse for a few times
3. Pour into pop molds and freeze for 2 hours
4. Serve and enjoy!

Nutrition (Per Serving)

- Calories: 155
- Fat: 15g
- Carbohydrates: 3g
- Protein: 2g

Dark Walnut Fudge

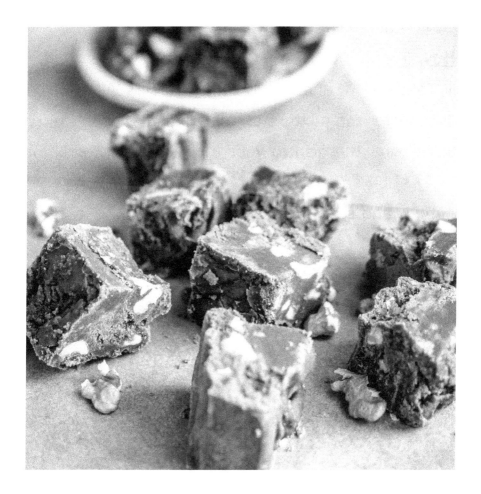

Serving: 4

Prep Time: 10 minutes

Ingredients

- 3 tbsp dark cocoa powder
- 4 and ½ oz of cream cheese, soft

- 1 and ½ oz of walnut pieces
- 1 tsp vanilla + 2 tbsp granulated sweetener
- 4 and ½ oz butter, soft

How To

1. Take a bowl and mix in all ingredients
2. Transfer the mixture to a lined dish
3. Transfer the dish to your fridge and let it chill for 2-3 hours
4. Slice and serve
5. Enjoy!

Nutrition (Per Serving)

- Calories: 124
- Fat: 12g
- Carbohydrates: 3g
- Protein: 2g

Keto Caramels

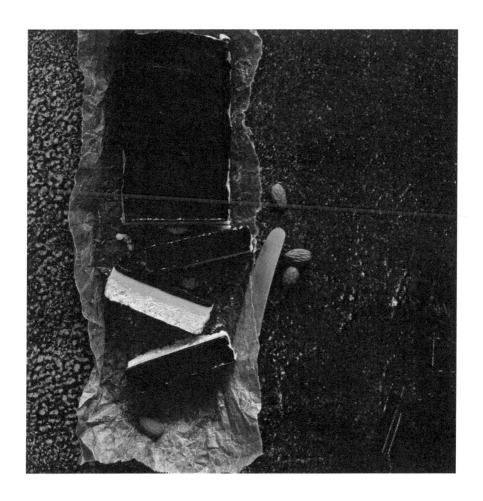

Serving: 4

Prep Time: 15 minutes + 3-4 Hours Chill Time

Cook Time: 5 minutes

<u>**Ingredients**</u>

- 2 c of heavy whip cream

- 6 tbsp of stevia powder extract
- 1 c of butter

How To

1. Take a non-stick saucepan and place it over medium-low heat
2. Add butter and let it melt, heat until light brown
3. Add cream and stevia to butter and paddle for 2 minutes until sticky
4. Remove from heat and keep mixing
5. Pour into candy molds and chill for 3-4 hours
6. Serve and enjoy!

Nutrition (Per Serving)

- Calories: 224
- Fat: 37g
- Carbohydrates: 2g
- Protein: 3g

Easy Vanilla Custard

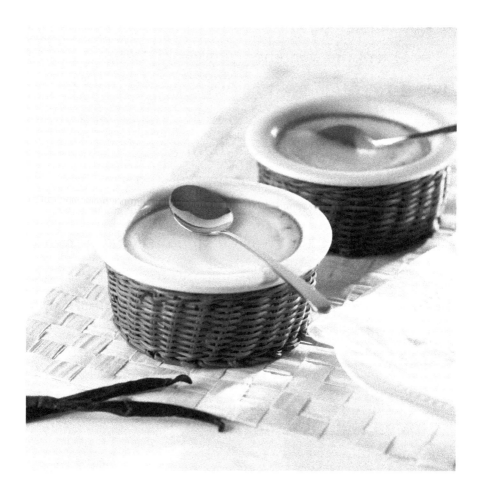

Serving: 4

Prep Time: 10 minutes

Cook Time: 5 minutes

<u>Ingredients</u>

- 1 tsp of vanilla extract

- 4 tbsp of melted coconut oil
- 1 tsp of stevia
- 6 whole egg yolks
- ½ c of unsweetened almond milk

How To

1. Whisk egg yolks, almond milk, vanilla, and stevia in a medium-sized metal bowl
2. Slowly mix in melted coconut oil and stir
3. Place the bowl over a saucepan of simmer water
4. Keep whisking the mixture vigorously until thick
5. Use a thermometer to register the temperature; once it has reached 140 degrees Fahrenheit, keep it steady for 3 minutes
6. Remove the custard from the water bath and serve chilled!

Nutrition (Per Serving)

- Calories: 197
- Fat: 15g
- Carbohydrates: 7g
- Protein: 5g

Raspberry & Coconut Barks

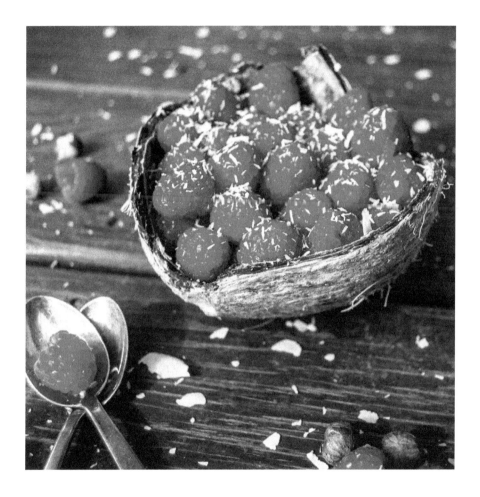

Serving: 4

Prep Time: 10 minutes + 60 minutes chill time

Ingredients

- ½ c of coconut butter
- ½ c of coconut oil

- ½ c of dried raspberries (frozen)
- ½ c of coconut, shredded
- ¼ c of swerve sweetener, powdered

How To

1. Power your frozen berries in a food processor
2. Keep the mixture on the side
3. Take a saucepan and place it over medium heat; add remaining ingredients and stir gently until melted
4. Pour half of the pan mixture into the baking pan (lined with parchment paper)
5. Mix in powdered berries to the remaining pan mixture and stir
6. Spoon raspberry mixture over coconut mix in your baking pan
7. Let it chill for 1 hour
8. Serve and enjoy!

Nutrition (Per Serving)

- Calories: 223
- Fat: 19g
- Carbohydrates: 5g
- Protein: 2g

Low-Carb Keto Angel Cake

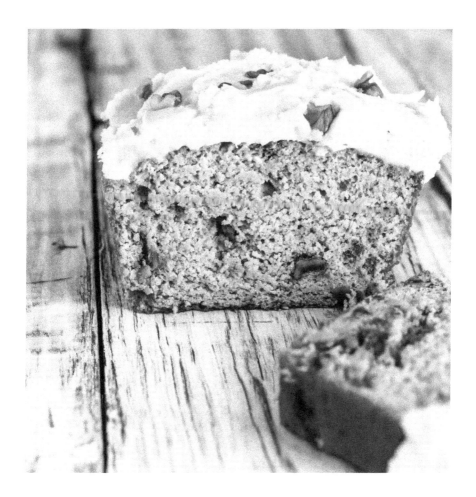

Serving: 4

Prep Time: 10 minutes

Cook Time:45 minutes

<u>**Ingredients**</u>

- 1 tsp of strawberry extract

- 12 egg whites
- 2 tsp cream of tartar
- 1 c of Egg white powder
- 1 c of powdered Erythritol

How To

1. Pre-heat your oven to 350 degrees F
2. Sift in whey protein, confectioners Erythritol and mix together
3. Take a large bowl and whip in egg whites, a pinch of salt, and mix until you have a foamy mix
4. Add cream of tartar, keep beating until very stiff and add your desired flavor extract
5. Quick fold in whey mixture
6. Pour the mixture into a 10-inch tube pan (greased) and bake for 45 minutes
7. Serve and enjoy!

Nutrition (Per Serving)

- Calories: 143
- Fat: 4g
- Carbohydrates: 5g
- Protein: 1.9g

Crust Free Mini Cheesecake

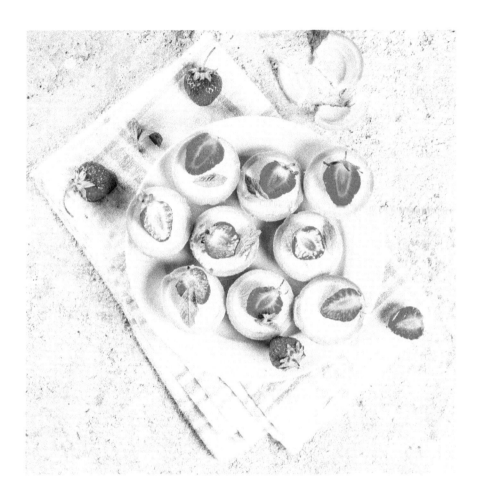

Serving: 4

Prep Time: 10 minutes + 3 hours chill time

Cook Time: 30 minutes

Ingredients

- 2 large whole eggs

- 1/3 c of natural sweetener
- ¼ tsp of vanilla extract
- 4 oz cream cheese
- ¼ c of sour cream

How To

1. Pre-heat your oven to 350 degrees F
2. Take a medium bowl and add cream cheese, sour cream, eggs, sweetener, vanilla and blend until thoroughly mixed
3. Place silicon liners in cups of a muffin tin
4. Pour the batter in your liners and bake for 30 minutes
5. Refrigerate for 3 hours
6. Serve and enjoy!

Nutrition (Per Serving)

- Calories: 159
- Fat: 13g
- Carbohydrates: 6g
- Protein: 2g

Jalapeno & Bacon Fat Bomb

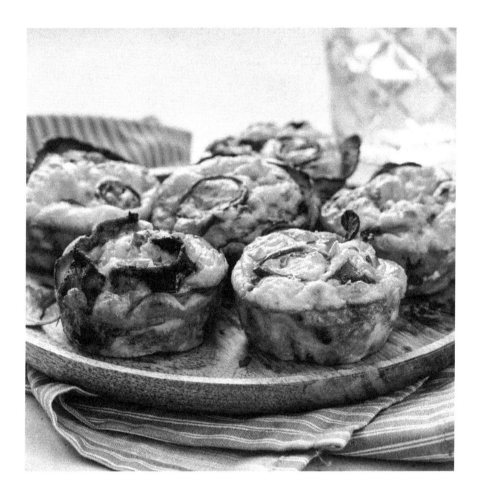

Serving: 4

Prep Time: 10 minutes

Cook Time: 10 minutes

<u>**Ingredients**</u>

- 6 ounces full fat cream cheese

- 2 teaspoons garlic powder
- 1 teaspoon chili powder
- 12 large jalapeno peppers
- 16 beef bacon strips

How To

1. Pre-heat your oven to 350 degrees Fahrenheit.
2. Place a wire rack over a roasting pan and keep it on the side.
3. Make a slit lengthways across jalapeno pepper and scrape out the seeds, discard them.
4. Place a nonstick skillet over high heat and add half of your bacon strip; cook until crispy.
5. Drain them.
6. Chop the cooked bacon strips and transfer them to a large bowl.
7. Add cream cheese and mix.
8. Season the cream cheese and bacon mixture with garlic and chili powder.
9. Mix well.
10. Stuff the mix into the jalapeno peppers and wrap raw bacon strips all around.
11. Arrange the stuffed wrapped jalapeno on a prepared wire rack.

12. Roast for 10 minutes.

13. Transfer to a cooling rack and serve!

Nutrition (Per Serving)

- Calories: 197
- Fat: 9g
- Carbohydrates: 8g
- Protein: 12g

Poppy Seeds Fat Bomb

Serving: 4

Prep Time: 10 minutes

Ingredients

- 8 ounces cream cheese, soft
- 3 tablespoons erythritol
- 1 tablespoon poppy seeds
- 1 lemon zest
- 2 tablespoons lemon juice
- 4 tablespoons sour cream

How To

1. Add listed ingredients to a bowl and mix using a hand mixer on low.
2. Once mixed, mix for 3 minutes on a medium-high setting.
3. Spoon mixture into mini cupcake cases and chill for 1 hour.
4. Enjoy once done!

Nutrition (Per Serving)

- Calories: 60
- Fat: 0.4g
- Carbohydrates: 2g
- Protein: 1g

Extremely Rich Choco Fat Bombs

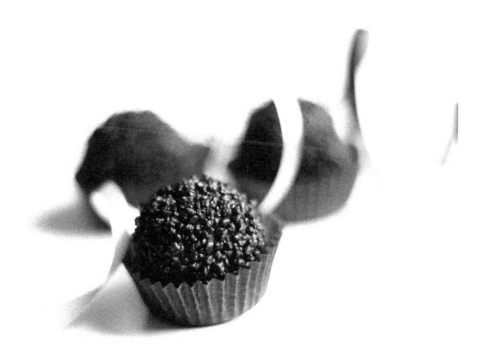

Serving: 4

Prep Time: 10 minutes + Chill Time

Ingredients

- 1 teaspoon vanilla essence
- 7 ounces heavy cream

- 5 ounces sugar-free chocolate
- 8 ounces cream cheese, soft
- 2 ounces icing mix

How To

1. Take a heatproof bowl and add water; let it simmer. Take another bowl and add chocolate; place bowl in simmer water to melt the chocolate.
2. Take another bowl and add cream cheese, use a hand mixer, and mix on medium speed until smooth.
3. Add icing mix and vanilla to the mix and mix on low.
4. Add heavy cream and mix on medium speed until thick.
5. Add melted chocolate to the mix and mix on medium.
6. Add mix to piping bag and pipe into cupcake tins, cover, and let them chill for at least 3 hours.
7. Serve and enjoy!

Nutrition (Per Serving)

- Calories: 87
- Fat: 8g
- Carbohydrates: 23g
- Protein: 1g

Fudgsicles

Serving: 4

Prep Time: 10 minutes + 60 minutes chill time

Ingredients

- 2 tablespoons cocoa powder, unsweetened
- 2 tablespoons chocolate chips, sugar-free
- 2 teaspoon natural sweetener
- ¾ cup heavy whip cream

How To

1. Blend the listed ingredients into your blender.

2. Blend until smooth.

3. Pour the mix into popsicle molds.

4. Keep in the fridge for 2 hours.

5. Serve and enjoy!

Nutrition (Per Serving)

- Calories: 199
- Fat: 19g
- Carbohydrates: 4g
- Protein: 2g

Chocolaty Bacon

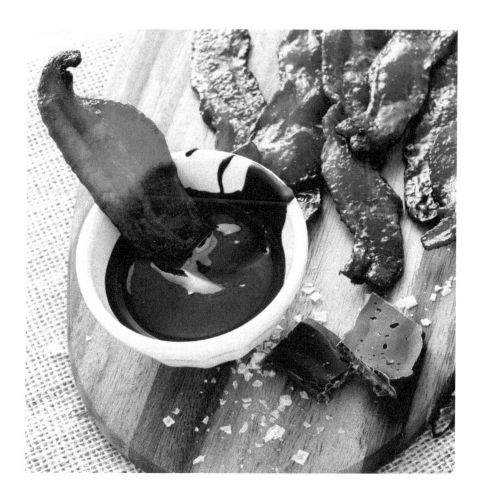

Serving: 6

Prep Time: 15 minutes

Cook Time: 20 minutes

Ingredients

- 2 and ¼ tablespoons coconut oil

- 1 and ½ teaspoons liquid stevia
- 12 beef bacon slices
- 4 and ½ tablespoons unsweetened dark chocolate

How To

1. Preheat your oven to 425 degrees F
2. Skewer bacon into iron skewers
3. Arrange skewers on a baking sheet and bake for 15 minutes until they show a crispy texture
4. Transfer to a cooling rack
5. Take a saucepan and place it over low heat, add coconut oil and let it melt
6. Stir in coconut chocolate and heat until it melts
7. Add stevia and gently stir
8. Place crispy bacon on parchment paper and drizzle chocolate mix
9. Let the chocolate harden
10. Serve!

Nutrition (Per Serving)

- Calories: 238
- Fat: 24g
- Carbohydrates: 1.5g
- Protein: 7g

Pink Yogurt Popsicles

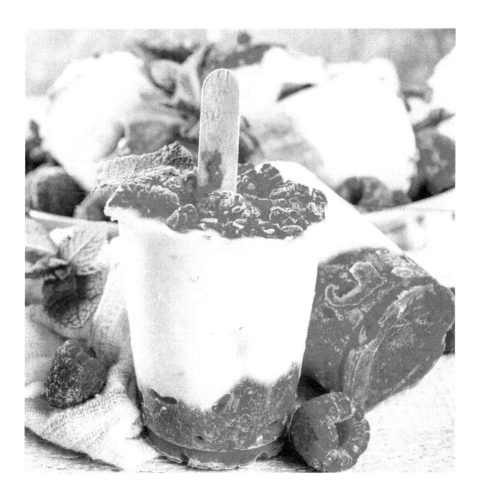

Serving: 4

Prep Time: 10 minutes + 3-5 hours chill time

<u>**Ingredients**</u>

- 1 cup Greek yogurt
- 2 and ½ teaspoons heavy whip cream

- 8 ounces frozen mango, diced
- 8 ounces frozen strawberries
- 1 teaspoon vanilla essence

How To

1. Blend the listed ingredients into your blender.

2. Blend until smooth.

3. Pour the mix into popsicle molds.

4. Keep in the fridge for 3-5 hours.

5. Serve and enjoy!

Nutrition (Per Serving)

- Calories: 192
- Fat: 18g
- Carbohydrates: 7g
- Protein: 5g

Lovely Pumpkin Buns

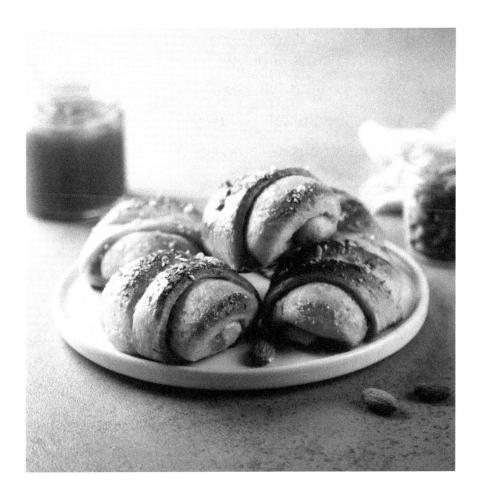

Serving: 10

Prep Time: 10 minutes

Cook Time: 50 minutes

Ingredients

- 1 teaspoon garlic powder

- 1 teaspoon baking soda
- 2 teaspoon cream of tartar
- ½ cup coconut flour
- 1 and ½ cups almond flour
- ½ cup ground flax seeds
- 1 teaspoon onion powder
- 5 tablespoons sesame seeds
- 1 teaspoons salt

Wet Ingredients

- 6 egg whites
- 1 cup warm water
- 1/3 cup Psyllium husk powder
- 2 Eggs

How To

1. Pre-heat your oven to 350 degree F

2. Take a baking tray and line it up with parchment paper, keep it on the side

3. Take a bowl and mix in dry ingredients, mix it well

4. Take another bowl and whisk in eggs, water and husk

5. Mix well until smooth

6. Slowly add dry ingredients into wet ingredients bowl

7. Keep mixing until you have an even dough

8. Knead dough until smooth and roll dough into buns, arrange them on your baking tray

9. Bake for 50 minutes

10. Once done, remove from oven and let them cool. Serve!

Nutrition (Per Serving)

- Calories: 179
- Fat: 12g
- Carbohydrates: 6g
- Protein: 10g

Gingerbread Keto Muffins

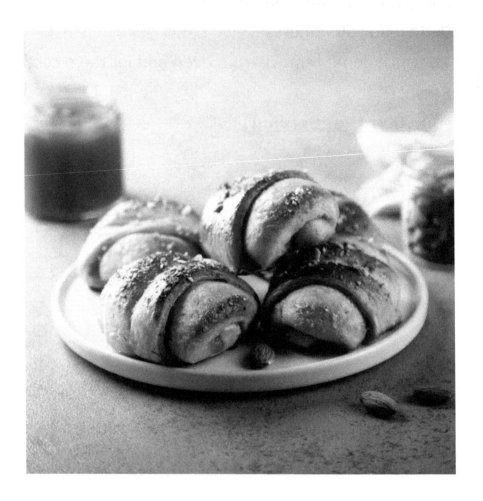

Serving: 6

Prep Time: 10 minutes

Cook Time: 10-15 minutes

<u>Ingredients</u>

- 1 tablespoon apple cider vinegar

- ½ cup peanut butter
- 2 tablespoons gingerbread spice blend
- 1 teaspoon baking powder
- 1 teaspoon vanilla extract
- 2 tablespoons Swerve
- 1 tablespoon ground flaxseed
- 6 tablespoons coconut milk

How To

1. Pre-heat your oven to 350 degree F

2. Take a bowl and add flaxseed, salt, vanilla, sweetener, spices and non-dairy milk

3. Keep it on the side

4. Add peanut butter, baking powder and keep mixing

5. Stir well

6. Spoon batter into muffin liners and bake for 30 minutes

7. Let them cool and serve

8. Enjoy!

Nutrition (Per Serving)

- Calories: 272
- Fat: 19g
- Carbohydrates: 11g
- Protein: 13g

Sensational Lemonade Fat Bomb

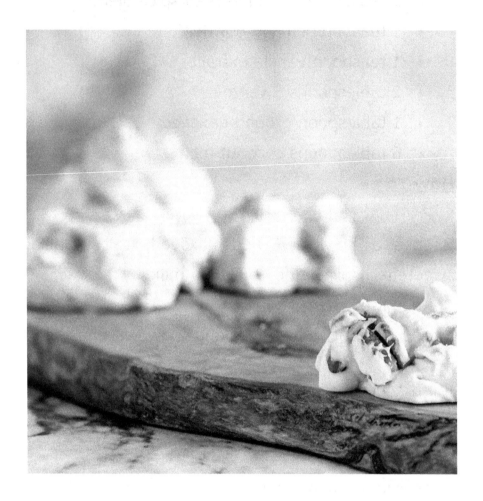

Serving: 2

Prep Time: 2 hours

Ingredients

- 2 ounces butter
- Salt to taste

- 2 teaspoon natural sweetener
- ½ a lemon
- 4 ounces cream cheese

How To

1. Take a fin grater and zest lemon

2. Squeeze lemon juice into bowl with zest

3. Add butter, cream cheese in a bowl and add zest, juice, salt, sweetener

4. Mix well using a hand mixer until smooth

5. Spoon mixture into molds and let them freeze for 2 hours

6. Serve and enjoy!

Nutrition (Per Serving)

- Calories: 391
- Fat: 39g
- Carbohydrates: 5g
- Protein: 4g

"No Bake" Fudge

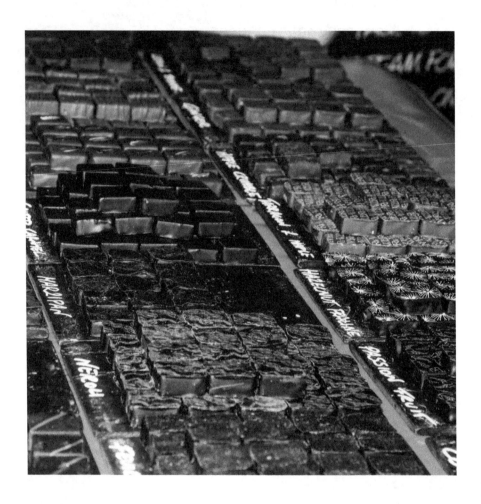

Serving: 25

Prep Time: 15 minutes + chill time

Cook Time: 5 minutes

<u>Ingredients</u>

- 1 teaspoon ground cinnamon

- ¼ teaspoon ground nutmeg
- 1 tablespoon coconut oil
- 1 and ¾ cups coconut butter
- 1 cup pumpkin puree

How To

1. Take an 8x8 inch square baking pan and line it up with aluminum foil

2. Take a spoon and scoop out coconut butter into a heated pan and allow the butter to melt

3. Keep stirring well and remove the heat once fully melted

4. Add spices and pumpkin and keep straining until you have a grain like texture

5. Add coconut oil and keep stirring to incorporate everything

6. Scoop the mixture into your baking pan and evenly distribute it

7. Place a wax paper on top of the mixture and press gently to straighten the top

8. Remove the paper and discard

9. Allow it to chill for 1-2 hours

10. Once chilled, take it out and slice it up into pieces

11. Enjoy!

Nutrition (Per Serving)

- Calories: 119
- Fat: 9g
- Carbohydrates: 5g
- Protein: 1.2g

Elegant Poppy seed Muffins

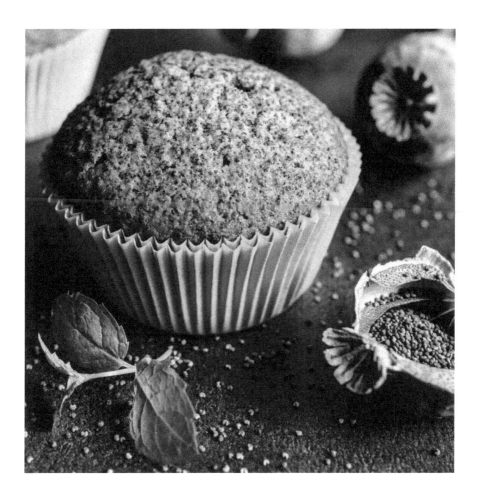

Serving: 6

Prep Time: 10 minutes

Cook Time: 10-15 minutes

Ingredients

- 1 teaspoon baking powder

- 2 tablespoons poppy seeds
- ¼ cup molted salted butter
- ¼ cup heavy cream
- 3 large whole eggs
- ¾ cup blanche almond flour
- ¼ cup golden flaxseed meal
- 1/3 cup Erythritol
- Zest of 2 lemons
- 3 tablespoons lemon juice
- 1 teaspoon vanilla extract
- 25 drops liquid stevia

How To

1. Pre-heat your oven to a temperature of 350 degree Fahrenheit

2. Take a mixing bowl and add poppy seeds, almond flour, Erythritol

3. Add the Flaxseed meal as well and let it stir completely

4. Add the melted butter

5. Pour heavy cream alongside egg

6. Mix everything well

7. Add baking powder, vanilla, lemon juice, stevia and zest

8. Mix everything to incorporate them well

9. Pour the batter into cupcake molds and bake for 20 minutes until a brown texture is seen

10. Cool the muffins on a cooling rack for 10 minutes and serve!

Nutrition (Per Serving)

- Calories: 279
- Fat: 29g
- Carbohydrates: 5g
- Protein: 2g

Swirly Cinnamon Muffins

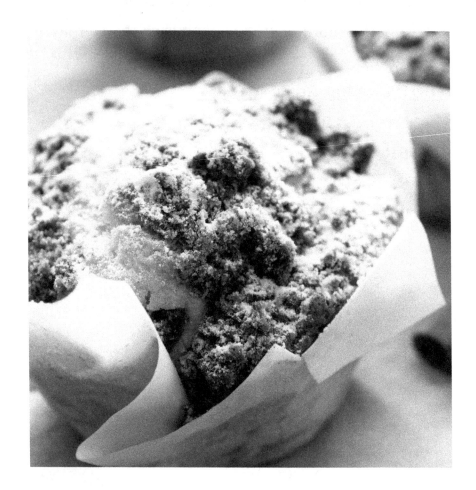

Serving: 6

Prep Time: 10 minutes

Cook Time: 10-15 minutes

<u>Ingredients</u>

- 3 egg

- 1 tablespoon coconut oil
- 4 teaspoons stevia
- 1 cup cauliflower, cooked and cooled
- ¾ cup Keto Friendly Protein Powder
- ½ cup ground peanuts
- 1 teaspoon baking powder
- 2 tablespoons Ghee, melted
- 1 tablespoon cinnamon

How To

1. Pre-heat your oven to 350 degree F

2. Grease muffin tin

3. Add cauliflower, peanut butter, powder, eggs, coconut oil, baking powder, stevia to a bowl and mix, keep it on the side

4. Pour batter into muffin tins

5. Take a bowl and add cinnamon and ghee, pour ½ teaspoon of the mix on top of each muffin and swirl using toothpick

6. Bake for 10 minutes

7. Remove from oven and let them cool

8. Serve and enjoy!

Nutrition (Per Serving)

- Calories: 410
- Fat: 24g
- Carbohydrates: 9g
- Protein: 33g

Mesmerizing Garlic Bagels

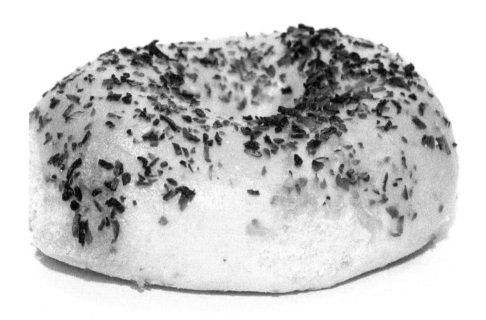

Serving: 6

Prep Time: 10 minutes

Cook Time: 15 minutes

<u>**Ingredients**</u>

- ½ teaspoon salt

- ½ cup coconut flour, sifted
- ½ teaspoon baking powder
- 6 whole eggs
- 1 and ½ teaspoon Garlic powder
- 1/3 cup butter, melted

How To

1. Pre-heat your oven to 400 degree F

2. Grease bagel pan and keep it on the side

3. Whisk in eggs, garlic powder, butter, salt to a bowl and keep it on the side

4. Add coconut flour and baking powder to egg mix, mix well until incorporated and a batter forms with no lumps

5. Pour batter into bagel pan

6. Bake for 15 minutes

7. Remove from oven and let them cool

8. Serve and enjoy!

Nutrition (Per Serving)

- Calories: 184
- Fat: 14g
- Carbohydrates: 6g
- Protein: 8g

Ravaging Blueberry Muffin

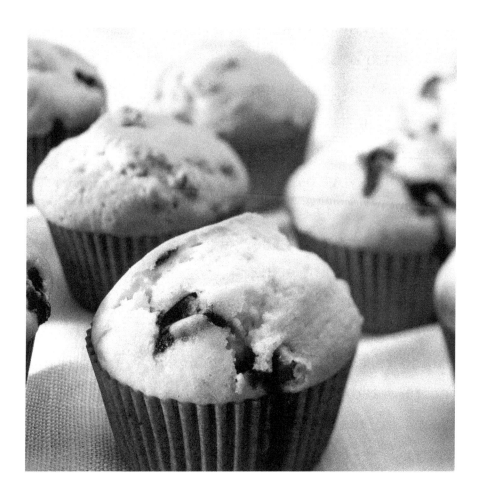

Serving: 4

Prep Time: 10 minutes

Cook Time: 30 minutes

<u>Ingredients</u>

- 1 whole egg

- 2 tablespoons coconut oil, melted
- ½ cup coconut milk
- 1 cup almond flour
- Pinch of salt
- 1/8 teaspoon baking soda
- ¼ cup fresh blueberries

How To

1. Pre-heat your oven to 350 degree F
2. Line a muffin tin with paper muffin cups
3. Add almond flour, salt, baking soda to a bowl and mix, keep it on the side
4. Take another bowl and add egg, coconut oil, coconut milk and mix
5. Add mix to flour mix and gently combine until incorporated
6. Mix in blueberries and fill the cupcakes tins with batter
7. Bake for 20-25 minutes
8. Enjoy!

Nutrition (Per Serving)

- Calories: 157
- Fat: 13g
- Carbohydrates: 1.7g
- Protein: 6.2g

No Bake Cheesecake

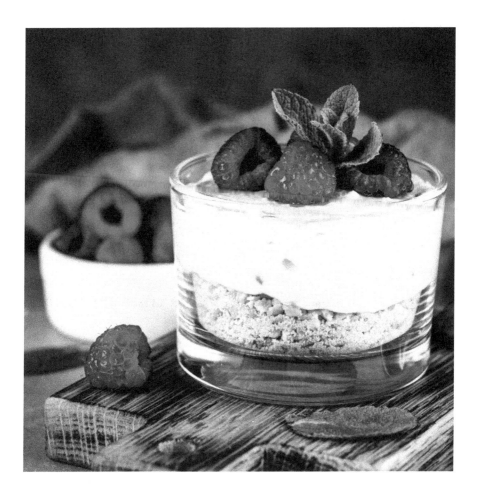

Serving: 10

Prep Time: 120 minutes

Ingredients

For Crust

- 1 teaspoon cinnamon

- 2 tablespoons ground flaxseeds
- 2 tablespoons desiccated coconut

For Filling

- ½ cup frozen blueberries
- 2 tablespoons coconut oil
- 1 tablespoon lemon juice
- 4 ounces vegan cream cheese
- 1 cup cashews, soaked
- 1 teaspoon vanilla extract
- Liquid stevia

How To

1. Take a container and mix in the crust ingredients, mix well

2. Flatten the mixture at the bottom to prepared the crust of your cheesecake

3. Take a blender/ food processor and add the filling ingredients, blend until smooth

4. Gently pour the batter on top of your crust and chill for 2 hours

5. Serve and enjoy!

Nutrition (Per Serving)

- Calories: 179
- Fat: 15g
- Carbohydrates: 5g
- Protein: 4g

Stylish Chocolate Parfait

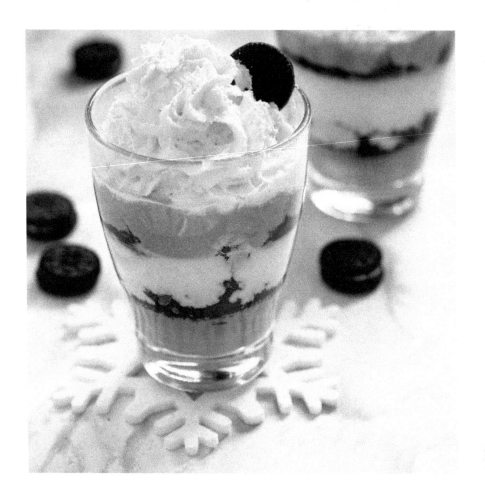

Serving: 4

Prep Time: 2 hours

Ingredients

- 1 tablespoon chia seeds
- Pinch of salt

- ½ teaspoon vanilla extract
- 2 tablespoons cocoa powder
- 1 cup almond milk

How To

1. Take a bowl and add cocoa powder, almond milk, chia seeds, vanilla extract and stir

2. Transfer to dessert glass and place in your fridge for 2 hours

3. Top with some berries, serve and enjoy!

Nutrition (Per Serving)

- Calories: 127
- Fat: 6g
- Carbohydrates: 8g
- Protein: 15g

Matcha Bomb

Serving: 10

Prep Time: 100 minutes

Ingredients

- 3/4 cup hemp seeds
- ½ cup coconut oil
- 2 tablespoons coconut butter
- 1 teaspoon Matcha powder
- 2 tablespoons vanilla bean extract
- ½ teaspoon mint extract
- Liquid stevia

How To

1. Take your blender/food processor and add hemp seeds, coconut oil, Matcha, vanilla extract and stevia

2. Blend until you have a nice batter and divide into silicon molds

3. Melt coconut butter and drizzle on top

4. Let the cups chill and enjoy!

Nutrition (Per Serving)

- Calories: 198
- Fat: 18g
- Carbohydrates: 4g
- Protein: 7

Almond Bread

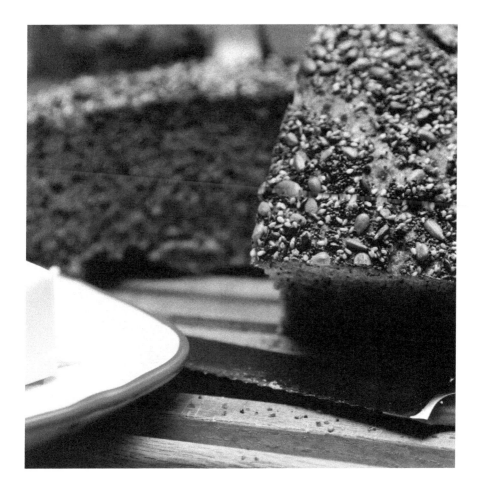

Serving: 8

Prep Time: 15 minutes

Cook Time: 60 minutes

Ingredients

- 3 cups almond flour

- 1 teaspoon baking soda
- 2 teaspoons baking powder
- ¼ teaspoon salt
- ¼ cup almond milk
- ½ cup + 2 tablespoons olive oil
- 3 whole eggs

How To

1. Pre-heat your oven to 300 degree F

2. Take an 9x5 inch loaf pan and grease, keep it on the side

3. Add listed ingredients to a bowl and pour the batter into the loaf pan

4. Bake for 60 minutes

5. Once baked, remove from oven and let it cool

6. Slice and serve!

Nutrition (Per Serving)

- Calories: 238
- Fat: 16g
- Carbohydrates: 6g
- Protein: 11g

Mesmerizing Avocado And Chocolate Pudding

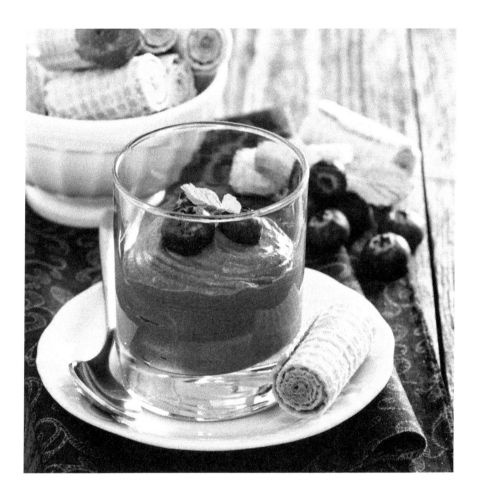

Serving: 2

Prep Time: 30 minutes

Ingredients

- 2 ounces cream cheese, at room temp

- ¼ teaspoon vanilla extract
- 1 avocado, chunked
- 1 tablespoon natural sweetener such as stevia
- 4 tablespoons cocoa powder, unsweetened

How To

1. Blend listed ingredients in blender until smooth

2. Divide the mix between dessert bowls, chill for 30 minutes

3. Serve and enjoy!

Nutrition (Per Serving)

- Calories: 277
- Fat: 23g
- Carbohydrates: 10g
- Protein: 8g

Great Fudge Popsicles

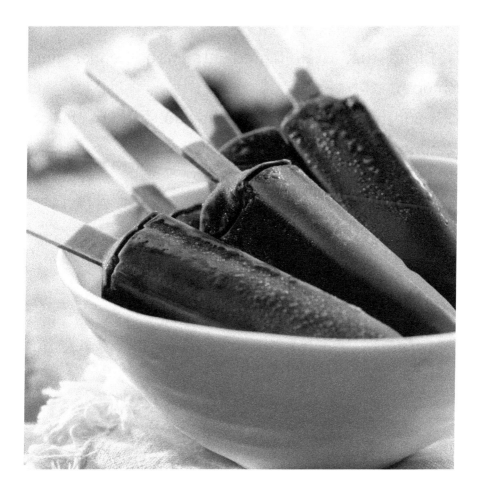

Serving: 4

Prep Time: 2 hours 5 minutes

Ingredients

- 2 teaspoons natural sweetener such as stevia
- ¾ cup heavy whip cream

- 2 tablespoons cocoa powder, unsweetened
- 2 tablespoons chocolate chips, sugar free

How To

1. Blend the listed ingredients in a blender until smooth

2. Pour mix into popsicle molds and let them chill for 2 hours

3. Serve and enjoy!

Nutrition (Per Serving)

- Calories: 188
- Fat: 17g
- Carbohydrates: 3.3g
- Protein: 2g

Egg & Coconut Bread

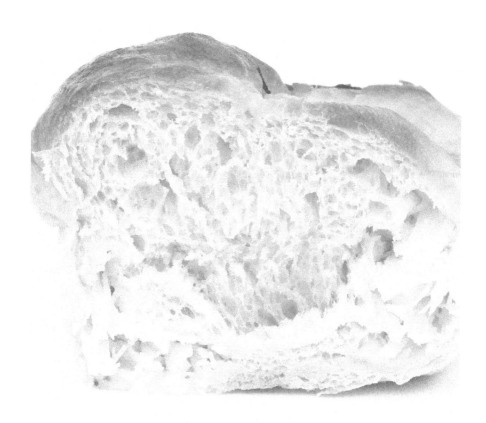

Serving: 4

Prep Time: 15 minutes

Cook Time: 40 minutes

<u>**Ingredients**</u>

- ¼ cup + 1 teaspoon coconut oil, melted

- ½ teaspoon garlic powder
- ½ cup coconut flour
- 4 whole eggs
- 1 cup water
- 2 tablespoons apple cider vinegar
- ½ teaspoon baking soda
- ¼ teaspoon Coarse salt

How To

1. Pre-heat your oven to 350 degree F

2. Grease a baking tin with 1 teaspoon coconut oil, keep it on the side

3. Add eggs to blender alongside water, vinegar, ¼ cup coconut oil, blend for half a minute

4. Add garlic powder, baking soda, coconut flour, salt and blend for a minute

5. Transfer to baking tin

6. Bake for 40 minutes

7. Serve and enjoy!

Nutrition (Per Serving)

- Calories: 291
- Fat: 12g
- Carbohydrates: 15g
- Protein: 16g

The Beasty Green Glass

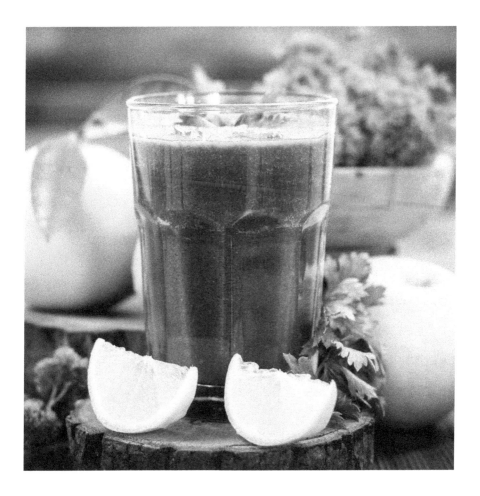

Serving: 1

Prep Time: 10 minutes

Ingredients:

- ½ avocado, peeled, pitted and sliced
- ½ cup frozen blueberries, unsweetened

- ½ cup unsweetened almond milk, vanilla
- ½ cup half and half
- 1 cup spinach
- 1 tablespoon almond butter
- 1 scoop Zero Carb protein powder
- 2-4 ice cubes
- 1 pack stevia

Directions:

1. Add listed ingredients to blender
2. Blend until you have a smooth and creamy texture
3. Serve chilled and enjoy!

Nutritional Contents:

- Calories: 255
- Fat: 15g
- Carbohydrates: 10g
- Protein: 17g

Spicy Bread Loaf

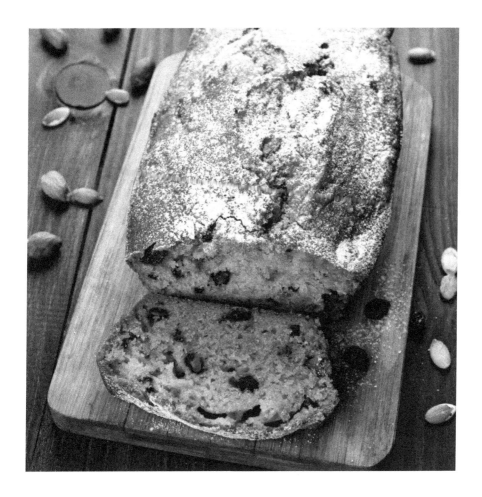

Serving: 4-6

Prep Time: 15 minutes

Cook Time: 55 minutes

Ingredients

- ¼ teaspoon salt

- ½ cup coconut flour
- 6 big whole eggs
- 3 big jalapenos
- 4 ounces turkey bacon
- ½ cup ghee
- ¼ teaspoon baking soda

How To

1. Pre-heat your oven to 400 degree F

2. Cut 3 big jalapenos and cut the jalapenos in slices, cut turkey bacon into thick slices

3. Place jalapenos and bacon on baking tray, roast for 30 minutes

4. Flip ad bake for 5 minutes more

5. Remove seeds from jalapeno and add jalapeno and bacon slices to food processor

6. Take a big bowl and add eggs, ghee, ¼ cup water

7. Mix well and add coconut flour, baking soda, salt and stir

8. Add jalapeno and bacon mix

9. Use a bit of ghee to grease the loaf pan

10. Pour batter into loaf pan

11. Bake for 40 minutes

12. Enjoy

Nutrition (Per Serving)

- Calories: 233
- Fat: 19g
- Carbohydrates: 6g
- Protein: 10g

Clean Sugar-Free Lemon Curd

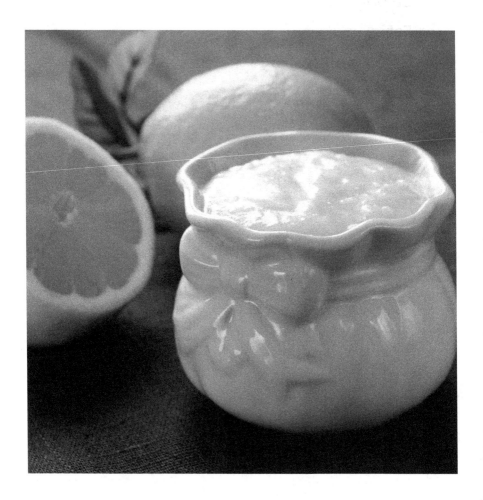

Serving: 2

Prep Time: 10 minutes

Cook Time: 10 minutes

Ingredients

- ½ cup grams of unsalted butter

- 3 whole eggs
- 1 egg yolk
- 4 unwaxed lemons (juice and zest kept)
- $1/3$ cup of erythritol or stevia

How To

1. Get a medium bowl and squeeze out the lemons and zest half of their skin.

2. Add the stevia or erythritol and the butter.

3. Heat a pan with boiling water and add the bowl with the lemon mixture on the toe (ben-Marie method). Careful so that the water doesn't touch the bowl.

4. Stir the mixture until the butter has melted.

5. Reduce to low heat and carefully whisk in the eggs. Keep constantly stirring and cook for 10 minutes. You should end up with a thin conditioner-like texture.

6. Remove from the heat and place on a sterilized jar or jars

Nutrition (Per Serving)

- Calories: 249
- Fat: 21g
- Carbohydrates: 3g
- Protein: 9g

Fantastic Hollandaise Sauce

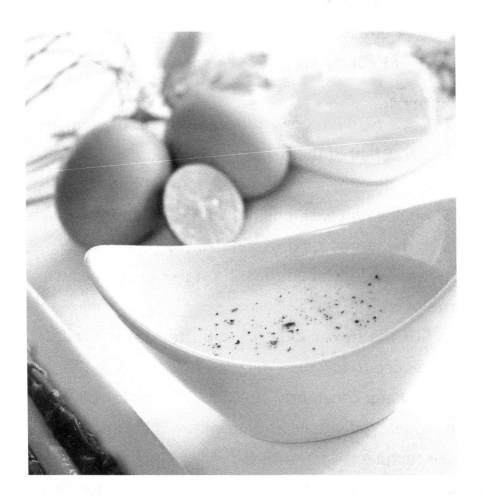

Serving: 4

Prep Time: 10 minutes

Cook Time: 1-2 minutes

Ingredients

- 2 tbsp fresh lemon juice 1 cup unsalted butter

- 8 large emulsified egg yolks $^1/2$ tsp salt

How To

1. Combine the egg yolks, salt, and lemon juice in a blender until smooth.

2. Put the butter in your microwave for around 60 seconds, until melted and hot.

3. Turn the blender on a low speed and slowly pour in the butter until the sauce begins to thicken.

4. Serve!

Mini Cheesecake Cups

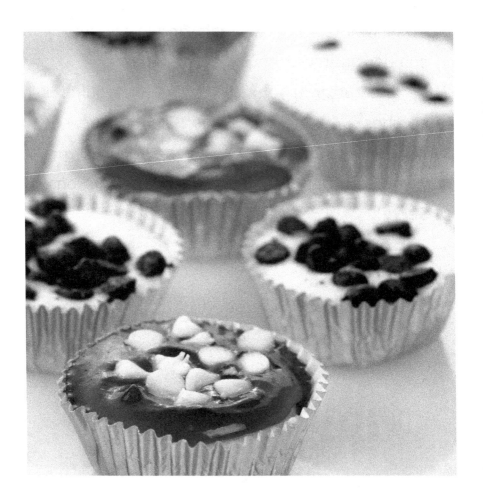

Serving: 4

Prep Time: 10 minutes + Chill Time

Ingredients

- 1 tsp Stevia Glycerite
- 1 tsp Splenda

- 1 tsp vanilla flavoring (Frontier Organic)
- 8 oz cream cheese, softened
- 2 oz heavy cream

How To

1. Combine all the ingredients.

2. Whip until a pudding consistency is achieved.

3. Divide into cups.

4. Refrigerate until served!

Nutrition (Per Serving)

- Calories: 245
- Fat: 17g
- Carbohydrates: 3g
- Protein: 7g

Raspberry Pudding Meal

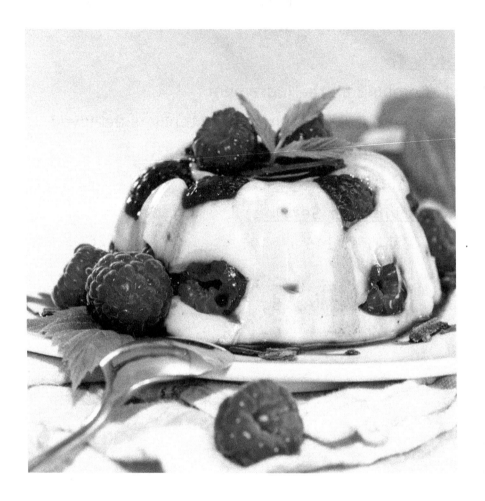

Serving: 4

Prep Time: 10 minutes + Chill Time

<u>**Ingredients**</u>

- 1 scoop chocolate protein powder
- $1/4$ cup raspberries, fresh or frozen

- 1 tsp honey
- 3 tbsp chia seeds
- $1/2$ cup unsweetened almond milk

How To

1. Combine the almond milk, protein powder, and chia seeds together.
2. Let rest for 5 minutes before stirring.
3. Refrigerate for 30 minutes.
4. Top with raspberries.
5. Serve!

Nutrition (Per Serving)

- Calories: 188
- Fat: 12g
- Carbohydrates: 12g
- Protein: 11g

Dreamy Vanilla Dessert

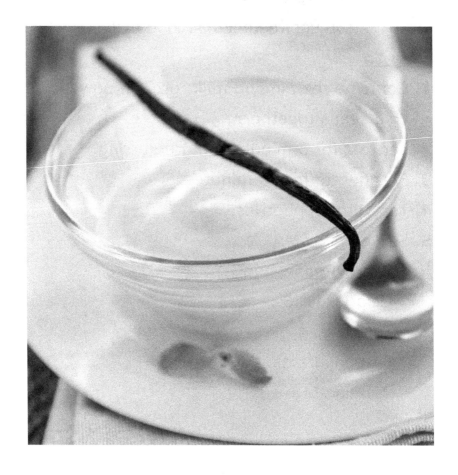

Serving: 2

Prep Time: 10 minutes +Chill Time

Ingredients

- Juice of 1 lemon
- Seeds from $^1/2$ a vanilla bean
- $^1/2$ cup extra virgin coconut oil, softened

- ¹/2 cup coconut butter, softened

How To

1. Whisk the ingredients in an easy-to-pour cup.
2. Pour into a lined cupcake or loaf pan.
3. Refrigerate for 20 minutes. Top with lemon zest.
4. Serve!

Nutrition (Per Serving)

- Calories: 197
- Fat: 15g
- Carbohydrates: 8g
- Protein: 9g

Cocopillow

Serving: 4

Prep Time: 10 minutes + Chill Time

Ingredients

- 1 can unsweetened coconut milk
- Berries of choice
- Dark chocolate

How To

1. Refrigerate the coconut milk for 24 hours.
2. Remove it from your refrigerator and whip for 2-3 minutes.
3. Fold in the berries.
4. Season with the chocolate shavings.
5. Serve!

Nutrition (Per Serving)

- Calories: 43
- Fat: 4g
- Carbohydrates: 3g
- Protein: 4g

The Brewed Coffee Surprise

Serving: 4

Prep Time: 10 minutes

Ingredients

- 2 heaped tbsp flaxseed, ground
- 100ml cooking cream 35% fat
- 1/2 tsp cocoa powder, dark and unsweetened
- 1 tbsp goji berries
- Freshly brewed coffee

How To

1. Mix together the flaxseeds, cream and cocoa, and coffee.

2. Season with goji berries.

3. Serve!

Nutrition (Per Serving)

- Calories: 49
- Fat: 33g
- Carbohydrates: 4g
- Protein: 17g

Crusty Almond Mini Cake

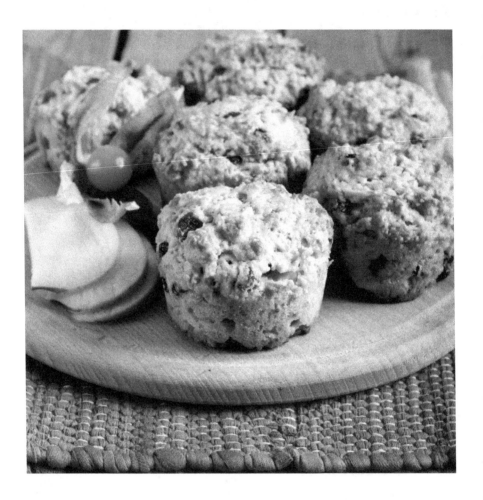

Serving: 4

Prep Time: 10 minutes

Cook Time: 30 minutes

<u>Ingredients</u>

- 1 cup keto almond flour

- 4 tsp melted butter
- 2 large eggs
- 1/2 tsp salt

How To

1. Mix together the almond flour and butter.
2. Add in the eggs and salt and combine well to form a dough ball.
3. Place the dough between two pieces of parchment paper. Roll out to 10" by 16" and $1/4$ inch thick.
4. Bake for 30 minutes at 350°F or until golden brown.
5. Serve!

Nutrition (Per Serving)

- Calories: 188
- Fat: 15g
- Carbohydrates: 4g
- Protein: 8.7g

Macaroon Bites

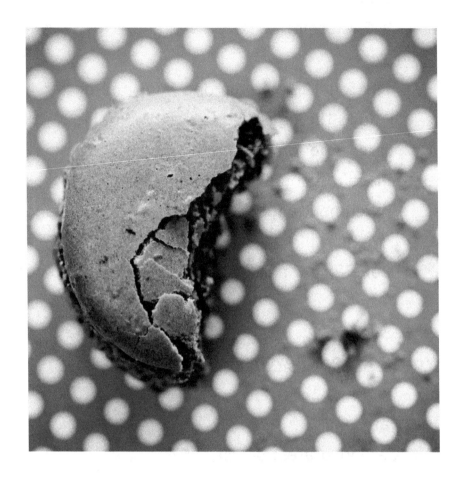

Serving: 4

Prep Time: 10 minutes

Cook Time: 15-20 minutes

Ingredients

- ½ tsp EZ-Sweet (or the equivalent of 1 cup artificial sweetener)

- 4 and 1/2 tsp water
- 4 egg whites
- 1/2 tsp vanilla
- 1 cup unsweetened coconut

How To

1. Preheat your oven to 375°F/190°C.
2. Combine the egg whites, liquids, and coconut.
3. Put into the oven and reduce the heat to 325°F/160°C.
4. Bake for 15 minutes.
5. Serve!

Nutrition (Per Serving)

- Calories: 119
- Fat: 11g
- Carbohydrates: 4.6g
- Protein: 3g

Chocolate & Coconut Pudding

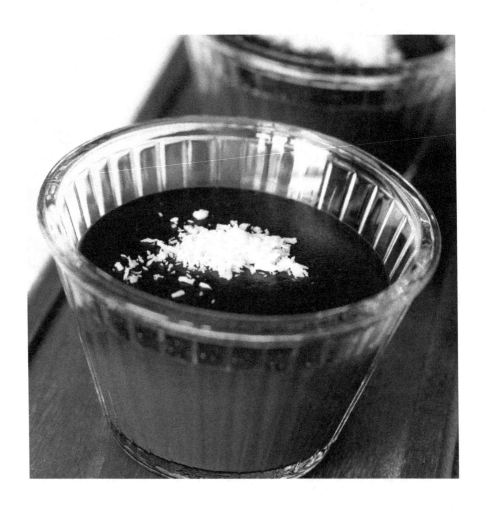

Serving: 4

Prep Time: 10 minutes + Chill Time

Ingredients

- $1/2$ tsp Stevia powder extract or 2 tbsp honey/maple syrup

- $1/2$ tbsp quality gelatin
- 1 cup coconut milk
- 2 tbsp cacao powder or organic cocoa
- 1 tbsp water

How To

1. On medium heat, combine the coconut milk, cocoa, and sweetener.
2. In a separate bowl, mix in the gelatin and water.
3. Add to the pan and stir until fully dissolved.
4. Pour into small dishes and refrigerate for 1 hour.
5. Serve!

Nutrition (Per Serving)

- Calories: 219
- Fat: 21g
- Carbohydrates: 5g
- Protein: 6g

Essential Chocolate Pudding

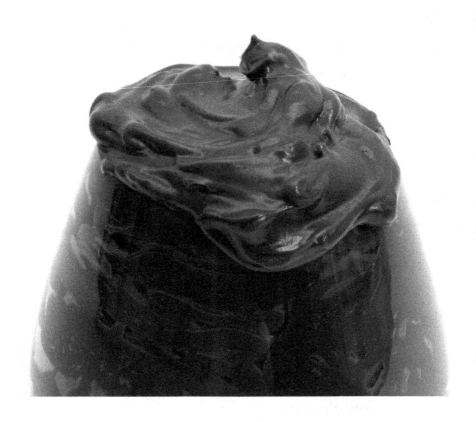

Serving: 4

Prep Time: 10 minutes + Chill Time

<u>Ingredients</u>

- 1 scoop cocoa powder
- $^1/4$ cup fresh raspberries

96

- $1/2$ tsp keto-friendly honey
- 3 tbsp chia seeds
- 1 cup unsweetened almond milk

How To

1. Mix together all of the ingredients in a large bowl.
2. Let rest for 15 minutes but stir halfway through.
3. Stir again and refrigerate for 30 minutes. Garnish with raspberries.
4. Serve!

Nutrition (Per Serving)

- Calories: 421
- Fat: 39g
- Carbohydrates: 6g
- Protein: 5g

Simple Cinnamon Cocoa Almonds

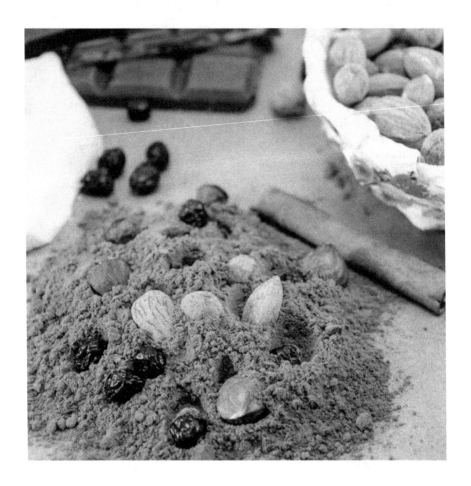

Serving: 8

Prep Time: 5 minutes

Cook Time:2 hours

Ingredients

- ¼ cup Erythritol

- 1 tablespoon unsweetened cocoa powder
- 1 tablespoon ground cinnamon
- 3 cups raw almonds
- 3 tablespoons coconut oil, melted

How To

1. Add almonds coconut oil to the slow cooker and stir until coated

2. Season with salt

3. Mix in Erythritol, cocoa powder, cinnamon, and cover

4. Cook on HIGH for 2 hours, making sure to stir every 30 minutes

5. Transfer nuts to a large baking sheet and spread them out to cool

6. Serve and enjoy!

Nutrition (Per Serving)

- Calories: 261
- Fat: 19g
- Carbohydrates: 6g
- Protein: 23g

Tip: *If you don't have a slow cooker, you may use an Iron-Cast Dutch Oven. The temperature is 200 Degrees F for LOW and 250 degrees F for HIGH*

Coconut Custard

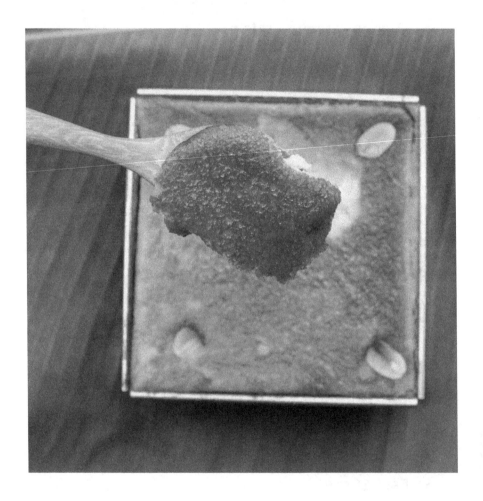

Serving: 8

Prep Time: 12 minutes

Cook Time:5 hours

Ingredients

- 1 teaspoon coconut extract

- 8 large eggs, lightly beaten
- 4 cups coconut milk
- 1 cup Erythritol
- 2 teaspoons stevia powder

How To

1. Coat the inside of your Slow Cooker with coconut oil

2. Stir in eggs, coconut milk, stevia, Erythritol, coconut extract to your Slow Cooker

3. Stir and place the lid

4. Cook on LOW for 5 hours

5. Let it cool for 1-2 hours

6. Serve and enjoy!

Nutrition (Per Serving)

- Calories: 375
- Fat: 35g
- Carbohydrates:4g
- Protein: 8g

Tip: *If you don't have a slow cooker, you may use an Iron-Cast Dutch Oven. The temperature is 200 Degrees F for LOW and 250 degrees F for HIGH*

Lemonade Fat Bomb

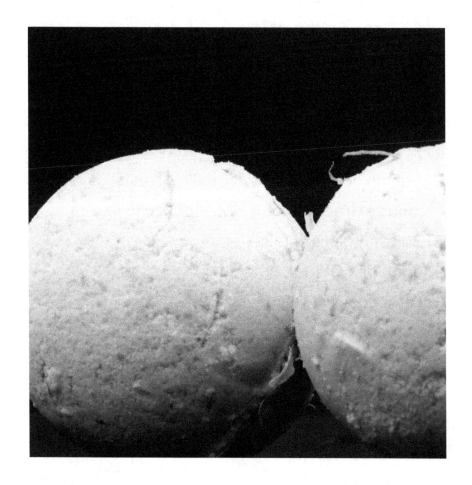

Serving: 2

Prep Time: 10 minutes

<u>Ingredients</u>

- 2 oz of butter
- 2 tsp of natural sweetener
- 1 whole lemon

- 4 oz of cream cheese

How To

1. Take a fine grater and zest your lemon
2. Squeeze lemon juice into a bowl alongside the zest
3. Add butter, cream cheese to a bowl and add zest, salt, sweetener, and juice
4. Stir well using a hand mixer until smooth
5. Spoon mix into molds and let it freeze for 2 hours
6. Serve and enjoy!

Nutrition (Per Serving)

- Calories: 397
- Fat: 39g
- Carbohydrates: 6g
- Protein: 5g

Chocolate Fat Bombs

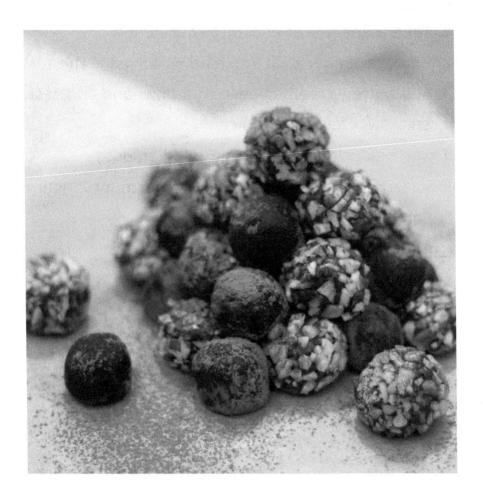

Serving: 4

Prep Time: 10 minutes + 1 Hour Chill Time

Ingredients

- 10 drops vanilla-flavored stevia drops
- ¼ c of coconut oil

- ¼ c of cocoa butter

How To

1. Take a small saucepan and place it over medium heat
2. Add coconut oil and butter, let it heat up until combined
3. Remove heat and stir in stevia until combined well
4. Pour mix into muffin tins and transfer to freezer
5. Let it chill for 1 hour
6. Serve and enjoy!

Nutrition (Per Serving)

- Calories: 309
- Fat: 18g
- Carbohydrates: 5g
- Protein: 11g

Vegan Spiced Fat Bomb

Serving: 4

Prep Time: 10 minutes + 90 Minutes Chill Time

Cook Time:

Ingredients

- ¼ c of hemp seeds
- ½ c of coconut oil
- 2 tsp of pumpkin pie spice
- 1 tsp of vanilla extract
- ¾ c of pumpkin puree

How To

1. Take a blender and add all of the ingredients
2. Blend them well and portion the mixture out into silicon molds
3. Allow them to chill and enjoy!

Nutrition (Per Serving)

- Calories: 98
- Fat: 9g
- Carbohydrates: 3g
- Protein: 1g

Keto Raspberry Chocolate Cups

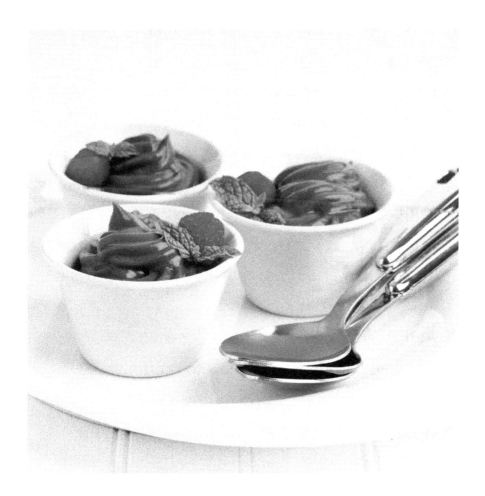

Serving: 4

Prep Time: 10 minutes + 60 minutes chill time

Ingredients

- 3 tbsp of granulated stevia
- 1 tsp of vanilla extract

- ¼ c of dried and crushed raspberries, frozen
- ½ c of cacao butter and coconut manna
- 4 tbsp of powdered coconut milk

How To

1. Prepare your double boiler to medium heat and melt cacao butter and coconut manna
2. Stir in vanilla extract
3. Take another dish and add coconut powder and sugar substitute
4. Stir the coconut mix into the cacao butter, 1 tablespoon at a time, making sure to keep mixing after each addition
5. Add the crushed dried raspberries
6. Mix well and portion it out into muffin tins
7. Chill for 60 minutes and enjoy!

Nutrition (Per Serving)

- Calories: 149
- Fat: 13g
- Carbohydrates: 2g
- Protein: 3g